The Story of Hemp

Panacea Life Sciences,

a Cannabinoid Company

LAUREN CAVARRA

LEARN MORE ABOUT PANACEA LIFE SCIENCES, INC.'S PRODUCTS AT WWW.PANACEALIFE.COM

CUSTOMER SERVICE AT 1 (800) 985-0515

Thank you to Lauren Cavarra for her hard work and authoring this book.

CONTENTS

A Brief History of Hemp

Quiz question: What was the first domestically-cultivated plant?

Time's up. If you picked up this book in the first place, you probably could guess that the answer is hemp, and you'd be correct. In fact, archaeologists argue that hemp was being cultivated as far back as 8,000 years ago in former Mesopotamia, and there are even pieces of evidence that could prove its cultivation an additional two or more thousand years earlier. Because of this, it's likely that hemp was the earliest plant cultivated for textile fiber, and it serves as the oldest example of human industry.

Hemp has played a tremendous role in the history of mankind. There are strong roots of hemp in China, which was the first country to recognize its use in paper production. Some of the oldest documents, Buddhist texts, were written on hemp paper that dates back to the second century AD. As it eventually made its way into Europe and the eastern Mediterranean by roughly 1,200 BC, hemp had become one of the most essential crops of the next several thousand years. By the middle ages, hemp was being made into rope and cordage, canvas for sails, clothing, fabrics, and more. While hemp had become vital to people's livelihood, nobody would have imagined that it would play a founding role in the rediscovery of the Americas.

In 1492, when Columbus sailed the ocean blue, the ropes and sails were rigged entirely from hemp fibers. While there are reports that hemp had already reached the continent before the Puritans took residence, early American farmers were quick to make use of the open land in order to grow hemp. Around the same time, King Henry VIII had begun to recognize the valuable trading and mercantile potential of the plant and mandated that all English farmers were to grow the crop or pay a fine. Shortly after this decree in England, the Virginia Assembly followed suit and ordered that "evr planter as soone as he may, provide seede of flaxe and hempe and sowe the same." Because of its profitable and seemingly endless uses, farmers throughout all colonies were legally required to grow hemp as a staple crop for the next several centuries. What's more, even the founders of our country were advocates of commercial hemp production; George Washington, Thomas Jefferson, John Adams, and Benjamin Franklin all grew and participated in hemp production. Thomas Jefferson is said to have drafted the Declaration of Independence on hemp paper (which has not been totally verified), and some historians claim that the 1776-made American Flag was fashioned from hemp. By the 1850s, the U.S. census registered approximately 8,400 hemp plantations, each producing at least 2,000 acres. Further north, hemp was grown throughout Canada long before confederation. hemp was seen as such a valuable crop that in the 1820s, Edward Talbot, Esq. noted, "if Canada produced enough hemp to supply Britain, it would end their dependence on foreign power and greatly benefit Canadian settlers."

[1]So, what happened? Cotton is certainly a partial entity to blame. Despite a 1916 report that found hemp to be capable of producing four times more pulp for paper manufacturing than traditional lumber sources, harvesting hemp was extremely labor-intensive. Towards the end of the 1700s, Eli Whitney's world-altering invention of the cotton gin was taking over, so naturally, people began to favor the production of cotton over hemp. By the time George W. Schlichten patented a hemp-processing machine in 1917, it was too late, and cotton had been established as the primary crop.

---

[1]   https://app.additor.io/p/UN4yjypt/a/2Q9H7dKB

Hemp's Bumpy Road

The Early 1900s

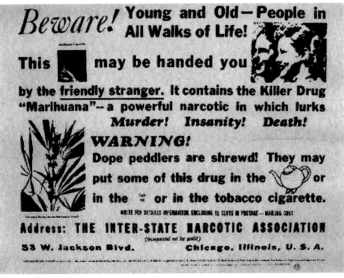

A 1935 U.S. government advertisement warning about dangers associated with marijuana. Origins.osu.edu

While many of us know the American 1920s as the "roaring twenties", filled with Prohibition-era speakeasies, flappers enjoying lavish parties, and romanticized images of gangsters and bootleggers, this decade was also full of culture clashes, consumerism, and politics based in fear. Of course, there was international instability caused by World War I and a fairly large agricultural slump, but most viewed it as an era of unprecedented, albeit lopsided, prosperity.[2]

Aside from automobiles, one of the most widely consumed products of the 1920s were radios, which found their way into more than 12 million households by the end of the decade. Radios became a beacon for family gatherings, where everyone would gather around to listen to the news, comedy shows, and music. In combination with newspapers, the rapid change in how quickly word could be spread and how many people it would reach would not only change the world as we knew it, but it would impact hemp production in a big way. More on this in a bit.

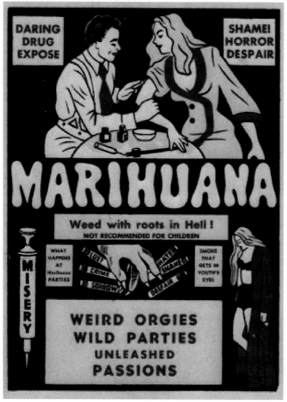

An ad for the 1930s film "Marihuana".
Credit: National Library of Medicine

2   https://www.history.com/topics/great-depression/1930s

Unfortunately, the prosperity of the 1920s couldn't last forever, and beginning in October of 1929, the United States experienced a decade-long economic downturn known as The Great Depression. 15 million Americans were left jobless, banks around the country crashed, investors were wiped out, and wide-spread panic became an unfortunate primary characteristic of people of the time. In the years where a lack of control turned into fear, fear turned into blame, and naturally, people across the country were seeking out someone or something to place that blame. Because the broadcast airways were largely run by prominent white men, one of many easy scapegoats were Mexicans who immigrated to the country in the early 1900s to seek refuge from the Mexican revolution. It became a widely-held belief that these immigrants were the first ones to present the use of cannabis for recreational purposes, so along with resentment of these people also came a negative connotation to what people referred to as "evil weed". Just like that, and riding on the heels of the Prohibition, by 1931, 29 states had made cannabis users outlaws.[3]

The most damning blow for the hemp industry was the fact that little was done to clarify the difference between cannabis products[4], so all strains from the plant cannabis were lumped under the one name of marijuana (then spelled as marihuana). As tensions rose within the country, the limited sources of information for the general public understandably became hard-held beliefs. Of course, some saw this as an opportunity to control and influence one of the strongest countries in the world for political and monetary gain, which is just what a man named William Randolph Hearst did. As the son of a gold-mine owner and U.S. senator, Hearst found his success as the owner of the *San Francisco Examiner* in 1887 and then *The New York Journal* in 1895. His successful ventures led him to some of the top positions in America, including serving in the U.S. House of Representatives (1903-1907)

---

[3]   https://www.ministryofcannabisblog.com/2018/03/22/marijuana-in-the-1930s-the-great-depression/

[4]   See Chapter 4.

and almost securing the title of the mayor of New York City. "By 1925, Hearst had established or acquired newspapers in every section of the United States, as well as several magazines. At the peak of his fortune in 1935, he owned 28 major newspapers and 18 magazines, along with several radio stations, movie companies, and news services."[5] With a virtual monopoly on news sources and communication, Hearst was privy to the amount of power he held. He also knew that his livelihood depended on the timber industry to support his papers, so naturally, hemp became his personal antagonist.

Hearst was not alone in viewing hemp as competition — namely, "the DuPont family, whose chemical company had just invented nylon and was allegedly afraid of competition from hemp fiber, [and] Andrew Mellon, Secretary of the Treasury and the nation's richest man, who had significant investments in DuPont".[6] As a final thrust in the war on hemp, John Rockefeller and Andrew Carnegie's financing of the rising pharmaceutical industry essentially sealed the deal. Together, these powerful forces were able to convince the general population of the United States that hemp was not only synonymous with immoral and nefarious commodities (like alcohol), but it also had incredibly negative connotations with Mexican immigrants. Playing on the fear of the American public, aggressive campaigns created effective propaganda in a time period we now look back on as the "Reefer Madness" era. With outlandish news stories, disturbing films, and sensationalized radio reports, any information available to the public falsely depicted cannabis as the most heinous drug on earth.

Ultimately, the US Government swiftly got involved, and in 1937, Congress passed the Marijuana Tax Act. The statute effectively criminalized marijuana, and because little was known about the difference between marijuana and hemp, the statute really criminalized the entire cannabis plant species.

---

[5]   https://www.britannica.com/biography/William-Randolph-Hearst
[6]   https://skeptoid.com/episodes/4401

The 1950s Through Early 2000s

The U.S. did see small resurgences of hemp and marijuana. In 1944 the New York Academy of Medicine issued an extensively researched report declaring that contrary to earlier research and popular belief, the use of marijuana did not induce violence, insanity or sex crimes, or lead to addiction or other drug use. Also, in the 1940's during World War II, imports of hemp and other materials crucial for producing marine cordage, parachutes, and other military necessities became scarce. In response the U.S. Department of Agriculture launched its "Hemp for Victory" program, encouraging farmers to plant hemp by giving out seeds and granting draft deferments to those who would stay home and grow hemp. By 1943 American farmers registered in the program harvested 375,000 acres of hemp. Then, in the 1950's and for decades to come, various anti-marijuana laws and stricter sentencing make it very difficult to experiment on and develop new uses for hemp, even with acknowledgement that hemp contains less than 0.3% THC, the plant's primary psychoactive ingredient.

Finally, the new millennium brought with the (re)enlightenment of hemp. Memorandums encouraging a more relaxed approach to enforcing the cultivation, distribution, sale and possession of marijuana were passed in 2009 and 2013. Then in 2014, two major events essentially jump-started cannabis's revival:

1. The federal court case Hemp Industries Association v. Drug Enforcement Administration (HIA vs DEA) has re-established acknowledgement of distinct varieties of Cannabis and supports the exemption for non-viable seed and fiber and any products made from them.

2. Colorado legalized marijuana for recreational use, followed closely by Oregon and Washington state.

As states continue to legalize cannabis products and more studies about its benefits are completed, the pendulum may swing in cannabis's favor for decades (hopefully more) to come.

The Farm Bill: Explained

In 2018, the contents of the Farm Bill contained a few essential provisions that would dramatically alter the legality and commercial landscape of Industrial hemp and Cannabidiol (CBD) forever. To understand what this bill did for CBD, let's look at a breakdown of the 2018 Farm Bill and the key takeaways for CBD.

Critical 2018 Farm Bill Benefit for CBD: Legalization

The biggest benefit that came from the 2018 Farm Bill is its order to remove hemp-derived substances from the controlled substances list. Prior to the bill, industrial hemp and any products derived from the hemp plant were considered dangerous and addictive drugs; law enforcement and community members even considered hemp products to be equivalent to heroin. Delisting CBD products effectively legalized CBD, so long as it comes from hemp that is legal under the Farm Bill itself.

Later chapters delve into the details about hemp and more specifically the differences between it and marijuana. For now, it's important to understand that hemp and marijuana are close relatives, but they are not the same. By definition, hemp contains no more than 0.3% THC — the psychoactive compound that is found in higher concentrations in marijuana. Marijuana products produce a high, whereas hemp products do not.

Circling back to the 2018 Farm Bill that legalized hemp, it's important to note that it more specifically legalized any subspecies of the Cannabis sativa L. plant with less than 0.3% THC (which means the legality of marijuana was not altered by the Farm Bill). Therefore, with the legalization of hemp, any derivative products that come from these plants (such as CBD) are also legal. As such, if the CBD is derived from the marijuana subspecies (that is, a plant with over 0.3% THC), then it is illegal to sell.

The Hemp Market is Not Entirely Free

Unfortunately, there are quite a few laws that intersect when it comes to cannabis and its legality. There are state laws as well as federal laws, and each level can conflict with another.

The 2018 Farm Bill is not a single comprehensive license to grow as much hemp as you want. It provides tight regulations that ensure that people are not able to grow hemp as freely as other crops like carrots and celery. In other words, this hemp bill won't let you buy a cannabis plant and put it in your backyard to grow CBD whenever you would like.

As previously stated, the Farm Bill does not, in any way, make cannabis with THC content above 0.3% legal. Federal law still classifies this as marijuana, and possession and growing marijuana carry steep penalties at the federal level. Therefore, you need to have a commercial enterprise where you can have 100% confidence that the plants you are growing will not have a THC content of 0.3% or above.

It is worth noting that laws are different from state to state. Medical marijuana is currently (as of 2020) legal in 33 states, and recreational marijuana is currently legal in 11. These states also have their own regulations on how cannabis may be grown and sold.

The other key piece to this legislation that restricts the hemp market is that it requires states to work with the United States Department of Agriculture (USDA) to create programs for licensing and regulating hemp. Only once the individual state has submitted their proposal to the USDA and the USDA approves that proposal can residents within that region produce industrial hemp. If some states don't want to create their own regulatory body, then people within those states can apply for a federally run program. Whether individual states create their own systems or residents have to opt-in to ones that the USDA has made, the reality is that growing hemp requires significant regulatory hurdles. Given all the hurdles and potential downsides for growing cannabis that may accidentally exceed 0.3%, it's clear that the market for growing hemp is not entirely "free". It's certainly less restrictive than before, but people will not be growing hemp in their backyards any time soon.

The 2018 Farm Bill Adds to Already Conflicting Laws

While the 2018 Farm Bill sought to bring clarity to the legal status of marijuana and hemp, it also added to the confusion. Part of the problem is that the laws at the state and federal levels often conflict in specific, intractable ways.

One way in which the laws intersect is with CBD-derived products. Currently, you can buy just about anything with CBD in it. From pain relief creams to oils to tinctures, manufacturers have been adding CBD to almost anything and everything, and new products and formulas are created all the time. Of course, there is a good reason for doing this. CBD has been reported to provide a multitude of health benefits from supporting joint health and flexibility to providing mental well-being. While the research into exactly how CBD accomplishes these outcomes is still in its infancy, it has been promising so far. Now, recall that the 2018 Farm Bill legalized CBD. Yet, in doing so, it legalized it in a very narrow manner. Any CBD-derived product created from industrial hemp, grown in full compliance with the Farm Bill itself, is legal. Technically-speaking, all this means is that CBD is no longer a Schedule I controlled substance. You cannot go to jail for possessing CBD extracted from a legal hemp plant.

However, this bill says nothing about how CBD products are to be regulated or manufactured. The Food and Drug Administration (FDA) has thus far issued unclear guidance regarding CBD products. The FDA is currently chiefly concerned about false claims being made by CBD companies and the language of health claims. As per the letter of the law, CBD cannot be added to a food product, but the FDA is not enforcing that rule particularly strictly. Furthermore, some states have expressly legalized CBD oil which makes it legal to sell within state lines, but despite these states' rules, federal laws still apply.

Ultimately, federal legality, state laws, and the FDA produce a legal compliance maze that leads to consumer and producer confusion. Even so, because of the popularity of CBD products, the reported positive health benefits, and the projected success of the CBD industry as a whole, lawmakers and regulatory agencies are working as rapidly as possible to clarify rules and regulations. The Farm Bill has been a great start, but there is much more work to do.

For the first time in half a century, the federal government was willing to decriminalize something – anything – related to marijuana. This decriminalization, even if it only applies to industrial hemp, represents a seismic shift in how politicians at this level view cannabis and its potential benefits.

There is already a growing body of research indicating that CBD may be a beneficial substance to improve overall human health. Ample research shows that CBD has potent anti-inflammatory properties, benefits for people (and animals) who suffer from anxiety or depression, may help with insomnia, may protect against neurodegenerative diseases, and may even promote heart health through its powerful antioxidant properties. In short, the body of research that shows CBD may be a true panacea for our bodies is growing.

While this bill did not explicitly legalize CBD from any source and in all forms, it did provide a legal pathway for researchers and consumers to obtain this impressive substance. That legalization is also forcing appropriate agencies, like the USDA and FDA, to have tough conversations to create a set of policy documents that are in line with the will of both Congress and the people. The fact that the bill removes CBD from the FDA controlled substance list is a hint to the other agencies to consider updating their rules and regulations appropriately.

The precise implications of the Farm Bill are still ongoing, however, the text within the bill is encouraging and may lead to more permissive CBD bills coming into law in the future, which we could see evidence of with the next Farm Bill in 2023.

FIVE Key Farm Bill Takeaways:

1. CBD derived from hemp containing less than 0.3% THC is now legal.
2. There are still restrictions on the production of industrial hemp.
3. The contradictory and murky laws are confusing.
4. The federal government's stance on marijuana (containing more than 0.3% THC) still has not changed.
5. The bill created newly opened paths for hemp research.

Government's Role in Hemp

Legality of CBD in the United States

CBD is legal in the United States — with certain restrictions. Which also means that it is available for purchase in most states. In 2018, a new version of the Farm Bill was passed. This is a bill that is reviewed, revised, and passed by the federal government every five years. The purpose of this bill is to lay out guidelines for all things agricultural, including what farmers can and cannot grow and sell. The 2018 version of the bill included a provision that legalized hemp.

The low level of THC in hemp is why it has been federally legalized; it's simply not enough THC for the psychoactive qualities to have any real effect. It's important to note that Marijuana is still federally illegal. However, a handful of states have legalized it. Some have only legalized the cannabis variation for medical use, while others have legalized it for recreational use as well. But what does this have to do with CBD?

Most CBD manufacturers prefer using hemp to extract the cannabinoid. This is because the high CBD levels and low THC levels makes the extraction process that much easier. When the 2018 Farm Bill was passed, it not only legalized hemp, it also effectively legalized any product made from hemp (as long as it is truly hemp-derived, containing less than 0.3% THC). This means that hemp products are legal across the country.

Should it be regulated?

The number of government organizations that influence the hemp industry is numerous including the United States Department of Agriculture (USDA) and Food and Drug Administration (FDA) to name a few. Navigating between three- and four-letter acronym agencies is no mean feat! Varying guidance or delays in regulatory decisions by both state governments and federal governments make it difficult to smoothly operate in this market sector. Seemingly small changes such as one state changing label requirements for hemp-based products creates operational complexity and cost increases. The uncertainty in regulation has major impacts (other than company headaches) on the hemp industry market potential which has been projected to be greater than $20B in a mere three years (Yahoo! Finance, Figure 2).

The Need for Regulatory Consistency for the Hemp Industry

Providing consistent guidance will allow farmers to determine the risks involved with growing hemp that include compliance as well as costs and profitability. Consumer product quality remains a very large issue with CBD products where over 75% products sold today do not meet potency requirements and may have THC levels beyond 0.3% (Bill J. Gurley, University of Arkansas, June 2019 presentation to the FDA; Rosemary Mazanet, Columbia Care, June 2019 presentation to the FDA). In addition to quality issues, CBD has been claimed to cure as many as 115 different conditions, some may be valid, others are wishful thinking. FDA guidance on how Phyto cannabinoid rich hemp products should be considered (food, supplement or drug) will provide standards on how products are produced, quality testing standards, consistent labelling requirements, as well as determine how research should be conducted to substantiate health claims.

Colorado has taken a unique approach of bringing together public and private stakeholders to modify the state regulatory environment through the CHAMP initiative (Colorado Hemp Advancement and Management Plan).

14

The CHAMP initiative evaluated the entire life cycle of the industrial hemp industry from seed to banking and marketing. While the full report and recommendations for regulations or legislation is due in Q2 2020, and will be discussed when the reports are published, it is important to understand that the CHAMP meetings have allowed progressive responses to proposed federal regulation.

USDA: Proposed hemp-growing regulations and the Interim Final Rule

Colorado, and other states, have worked for the past five years under the regulatory system enabled by the 2014 Agriculture Improvement Act, also known as the Farm Bill. In this bill, hemp could be grown under a pilot program with guidance on how the states should regulate the growth of hemp. The 2018 version of the Farm Bill effectively moved hemp and hemp-based products out of a pilot phase and called for the USDA to develop a final regulatory plan for farming industrial hemp. The initial USDA plan termed the Interim Final Rule (IFR) was published with a request that individual states provide comments and submit their own plans on how they would comply with USDA regulations. Understanding the implications of how the regulations proposed in the IFR will affect hemp growers is extremely important. In Colorado's response to the USDA IFR, Colorado has asked the USDA to extend the 2014 growing rules for another year to ensure better understanding of the proposed rule changes and arrive at a balance between protecting public health and healthy hemp farming industry. Quite frankly, it is disappointing that states without significant numbers of hemp farmers have adopted the IFR as written without critical consideration of impact. To directly quote a Colorado state senator, "The regulations proposed in the IFR will kill the hemp industry." Colorado, being the largest producer and having the longest tenure in growing hemp has assembled a very thoughtful and data driven response to the IFR. Two major highlights of the plan and why suggested changes be made to the IFR are listed below. The link to Colorado's response to the IFR is located on their site and will provide a more detailed and complete explanation of the impact to the IFR and what changes are suggested. Note that the response to the USDA was supported by the Colorado State Senate resolution 20-005 with overwhelming support.

Sampling periods and coverage.

The IFR calls for 100% of the registered hemp fields be tested at DEA approved laboratories prior to harvest. In addition, the crop is to be completely harvested 15 days after sampling. This will have the highest concentration of cannabinoids in the plant. Additionally, there is a 15 day period from when the sample is submitted to when the fields must be harvested with harvest prior to receiving test results prohibited.

Please note that the sample takes the flower from the top 2-6" of the plants free of stem, leaves and seed constitute the tested sample.

In 2019, Colorado had 87,000 acres registered to plant hemp through 2,600 growers. Under Colorado's state plan, harvest can occur within a 30-day window after sampling. Employing a random sampling Colorado 23% (619 registrants, 2,712 lots) were evaluated. Using the proposed IFR rules would create a large bottleneck and resource constraint where the state laboratory would need to expand by at least four-fold to meet testing demands and seek DEA registration for hemp laboratories. Needless to say, the IFR rules would create delays in the time farmers could harvest which puts more risk on the crop due to weather variations, especially in Rocky Mountain states.

Colorado has recommended that there be a 30-day period between sampling and harvest, consider random sampling, and eliminate the DEA laboratory requirement so that state laboratories with appropriate standards (ISO17025) can continue testing for crop compliance.

Table A. Colorado Hemp Test Result Distribution

2019 THC Test Results*	2019 Colorado Data				Scaled to 100% Sampling Coverage			
	Producers	Registrations	Acres**	Total Economic Value	Producers	Registrations	Acres**	Total Economic Value
<= 0.3	369	398	11,800	$405,413,512	1,276	1,694	64,568	$2,217,109,996
> 0.3%	209	221	4,491	$154,460,821	723	940	24,529	$842,923,678
> 0.4%	98	102	2,654	$91,226,304	339	434	14,492	$497,742,332
> 0.5%	45	48	1,560	$53,574,180	156	204	8,512	$292,254,674
> 1.0%	11	11	289	$9,945,697	38	47	1,579	$54,248,178

Notes: * Each figure for producers, registrations, etc. is cumulative and includes all samples that tested above the THC test result value in the left column. We assume that the distribution of test results for 100 percent of registrations would be the same as observed in 2019 actual testing.

        **Reported acreage includes all indoor hemp cultivation, scaled from square feet to acres.

Source: CDA; USDA; MPG Consulting LLC.

Thresholds for Destruction and Negligence

Since 2014 Colorado has destroyed over 3,360 acres of hemp worth roughly $115,000,00, in total, due to the hemp testing above 0.3%. If the IFR requirements of 100% testing at the 0.3% level were implemented for the 2019 harvest, the estimated acres that would need to be destroyed is estimated at 24,500 with an economic value of $842,600,000.

Colorado has proposed several possible methods for helping avoid destruction of these crops that protects the industry against bad actors yet allows use of crops that test above 0.3% in the sampling period. As stated above, the sampling takes the uppermost flower from the plant which will have the highest cannabinoid concentration. Three simple changes would be to allow post-harvest testing, increase the destruction threshold to 1% and allow non-compliant hemp to enter a THC-remediation program where extractor/processors would remove THC from the extracted oil so that only 0.3% THC products would then be able to be sold.

Typically, hemp is sold to processors as a whole plant homogenate that is a mixture of flowers, leaves and stems. Since the leaves and stems of the plant contain very small amounts of cannabinoids, a plant that tests slightly higher than 0.3% would be compliant when turned into homogenate. Elevating the threshold and requiring any crops that still test higher than 0.3% and <1% to enter a remediation program at reduced costs allows the farmer to recover costs and ensures that deviate from industrial hemp definitions be commercialized. Implementation of these changes would have lead to 1% of Colorado's hemp crop to be destroyed for non-compliance.

Setting the threshold at 1% THC for negligent violations verses 0.5% would mitigate grower risk due to some uncertainties in crop growing conditions and allow a more efficient industry. Under the IFR rules, 48 negligent violations would be issued, as opposed to 11 if a 1% threshold was adopted. Non-compliant hemp, regardless of the threshold set, should be allowed to be destroyed by the farmer on-site under the supervision of state or tribal agriculture departments. Moving this threshold balances the need to protect public health and facilitate the development of a thriving hemp industry.

FDA: Is CBD safe; should industrial hemp oil be a food ingredient, dietary supplement or drug?

As clearly stated in the 2018 Farm Bill the FDA has oversight of products derived from industrial hemp. Although there have been many meetings and conversations by the FDA and the public, progress is moving at a glacial pace. The new commissioner, Stephen Hahn understands that the toothpaste is out of the tube so the situation needs to be managed: "We're not going to be able to say you can't use these products. It's a fool's errand to even approach that [.] We have to be open to the fact that there might be some value to these products and certainly Americans think that's the case. But we want to get them information to make the right decisions." The FDA just opened the public comment and invitation for submission of data for clarifying the points listed below, but has yet to lay out a definitive pathway for regulation of CBD-containing products. The March 2020 report to the congressional appropriations committees provides insight as to the FDA focus and goals for the coming year. While the FDA is exploring how various CBD products can be lawfully marketed, is very concerned about potential safety risks, mislabeling products, and that the products contain contaminants such as delta-9 tetrahydrocannabinol (THC), heavy metals and pesticides as there are no manufacturing standards. The FDA recognizes that research has been restrictive until the farm bill passed so is inviting all data submissions from public and private entities, reaching out to state health departments as well as ensuring there are incentives for performing clinical research. What has been needed is exactly what concerns the FDA has so that researchers can design studies to answer those questions definitively.

The key questions the FDA is seeking to address:

1. What happens if you use CBD daily for sustained periods of time?
2. What level of intake triggers the known risks associated with CBD?
3. How do different methods of exposure affect intake (oral, topical, smoking or vaping)?
4. What is the effect of CBD on the developing brain?
5. What are the effects of CBD on an unborn child or breasted newborn?
6. How does CBD interact with herbs and botanicals?
7. Does CBD cause reproductive toxicity in males?
8. Are there different safety concerns for use in certain animal species, breeds or classes?
9. Are any residues formed in edible tissues of food producing animals?

In addition to these questions, the FDA is seeking more information on identity standards on varying CBD products such as full-spectrum or broad-spectrum oils and how these products are derived. A grant has been awarded to study CBD effects on fetal growth in pregnant women, and has launched an initiative with the University of Mississippi to sample commercial CBD products to determine CBD and THC levels in 100 cosmetic products as well as dermal penetration that is intended to be published in August, 2020.

In the 2020 report, the FDA reiterates priorities focused on determining safety, enforcement of products making disease claims, and ensuring product potency and purity. Currently the FDA has stated that it is illegal to introduce CBD into human or animal food, market as a dietary supplement, and CBD may be illegal in cosmetics if intended to affect structure/function or address a disease. Minor cannabinoids CBG and CBN have been mentioned as well that raise concerns about claims and safety. It is very important to note that the FDA considers CBD a schedule V drug due to clinical trials beginning on Epidiolex prior to CBD being marketed. While these statements have been repeated by the FDA over the past three years there is cause for optimism for hemp growers, manufacturers and consumers. The FDA is actively considering potential pathways for certain CBD products to be marketed as dietary supplements. Additionally, the report states that the FDA has the authority to create an exemption through notice and public comment.

While the report gives better insight as to the focus and plan moving forward, it is very puzzling on why more progress has not been made. As stated above, the main focus of the FDA is whether these compounds are safe. One could argue that there is a wealth of information that can be compiled to answer these concerns with any additional concerns being addressed by specific studies with defined timelines. In contrast to the glacial pace of FDA progress, CBD regulatory pathways have been established in the UK, Germany, and it has been approved by the World Health Organization (WHO).

There have been 226 CBD clinical studies registered with the federal government, with over 80 studies completed. These studies have administered CBD to patients at doses as high as 40 mg/kg/day. Each study reports on clinical efficacy as well as side effects. Since one requirement to enter into a clinical study is safety, it is puzzling how these clinical studies could be approved, yet there are so many safety concerns stated in the 2020 report. In a <u>2018 report WHO</u> states that CBD is generally well tolerated with a good safety profile as well as not demonstrating any public health related problems. The report states that at common consumption levels CBD is fundamentally safe. The <u>Food Standards Agency</u> (FSA), the agency that regulates CBD in the United Kingdom, has approved CBD at a 70 mg per day serving unless under medical supervision. The CBD products must contain <0.01% THC and have no other controlled cannabinoid such as Tetrahydrocannabivarin (THC-V). The FSA does state that they wish there was more safety data with pregnant women and drug-drug interactions, but this agency has laid out specific regulatory requirements with all producers to comply by March 31,

2021. Germany has followed suit allowing CBD to be a food ingredient. This raises the question on why the FDA has not taken a similar approach?

Due to the lack of significant progress by the FDA, both public and private groups are working to obtain regulatory clarity. At the federal level, HR5587 is a bill submitted to the house of representatives by congressman Comer (MN) to put into law that CBD is an exception to the IND rule stated above and that this product be regulated as a dietary supplement. Utah has issued a resolution SCR11 that "Urges the Issuance of Federal Guidelines to Protect Consumers of Cannabidiol Products" which has been sent to the President and leaders of the house or representatives and senate. Private initiatives are forming coalitions to engage the FDA to obtain progress. Validcare has launched an industry-sponsored CBD liver safety study with a goal of monitoring chronic CBD usage at varying doses on liver function. This study will enroll up to 2000 patients with data reported in September, 2020. The National Industrial Hemp Council is forming a Consumer Protection Task Force comprised of over 20 subject matter experts to focus on outstanding issues stated by the FDA and engage the FDA's CBD working group. This approach may be very productive to address specific issues to responsibly accelerate progress towards how CBD will be regulated.

The Impact of the Lack of Regulatory Framework

As stated in the opening of this document, the rules or lack thereof, create a maze that changes constantly yet needs to be navigated to produce quality products and meet consumer demand. It may seem like an oxymoron pairing the need for regulatory rules with economic success, but the reality is that the lack of clarity by the FDA has stifled the economic potential of the hemp industry by allowing consumer confusion and in effect restricting retail markets. Similarly, not having a usable framework for growing hemp and processing into oil as a manufacturing ingredient has had a negative impact on farmers.

Both the FDA and private companies need to reach an agreement on standards of identity. The definition and criteria for various preparations of CBD vary within the industry. Consumers do not understand what a full-spectrum, broad-spectrum, or isolate product is and what benefits or risk they may obtain with each product. Similarly, there are not uniform manufacturing standards that all CBD product are held. The result is that many products do not meet potency or purity that are standard in the food and dietary supplement industry. The result of confusion and inferior products on the market create mistrust by consumers which causes lower demand.

There has been an expectation that following the passing of the 2018 Farm Bill that there would be clear regulations on how hemp would be grown, products would be manufactured, labelled and sold to consumers. Consumers understand that there are numerous health benefits provided by CBD but manufacturers do not know how they should label products or educate consumers without receiving a warning letter from the FDA. Likewise, retail outlets have held off on carrying CBD products as they need to understand where these products should be placed, how they can market, and do not want to face product confiscation or recalls. The lack of clarity has significantly impacted CBD sales. Market forecasts as shown in Figure 1 below has projected the US CBD to exceed $20 billion dollars by 2022. The current 2020 CBD revenue projection is hopefully going to reach 20% of forecast as shown in Figure 2.

The hardest hit with the market not reaching anywhere close to expectations are the hemp farmers. Since hemp is grown like any other commodity, acres grown are planned in the early summer with the hope and expectation that the crop will be purchased at reasonable market rates. Hemp is normally sold at dollars per percentage point per pound (PPPP). Thus, a 10% CBD crop sold at $5 PPPP would be $50 per pound. The 2018 crop production met existing demand with a range of pricing from $3.5 PPPP to $7.5 PPPP. Heading into the 2019 growing season farmers scaled up production that exceeded usable demand causing hemp prices to plummet. Without clarity to expand retail markets, the anticipated demand was not realized. It is striking to map hemp prices following FDA statements as shown in Figure 3. Clearly, prices realized by the farmers correlates to continued lack of clarity by the FDA.

Figure 1: US Hemp CBD Market Forecast by year

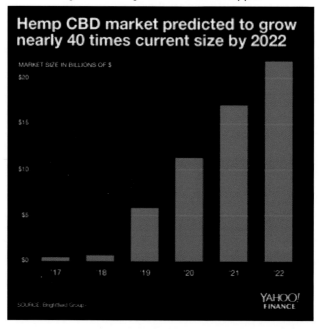

Figure 2: Actual US CBD revenue and projected 2020 revenue by CBD source

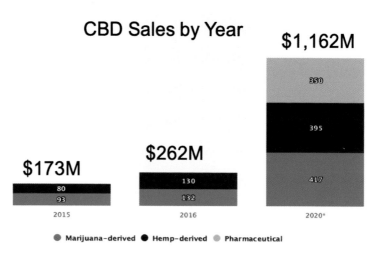

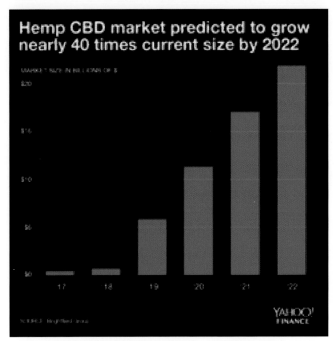

Figure 3: FDA statement correlation to US Hemp prices

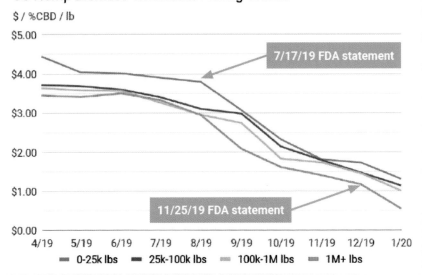

Source: Hemp benchmarks: https://hempbenchmarks.com

All About the Hemp (Cannabis) Plant

Note: The official classification of Cannabis is still unclear. "The naming conventions for Cannabis sativa and Cannabis indica are still debated to this day. Some experts believe there is only one species of Cannabis, Cannabis sativa L., with three distinct subspecies. Still other experts believe that cannabis sativa and cannabis indica are their own separate species." (The Universal Plant). Going forward in this book, we will use the classification shown in the image below.

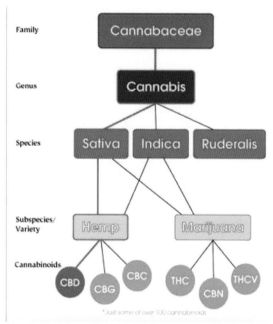

In order to fully understand the relationship between hemp (from which CBD is extracted) and marijuana, let's start by looking at the source of each:

Cannabis Sativa L. There are many cannabinoids found in the Cannabis sativa plant, which is why THC and CBD are often confused with one another. However, they are very different. While hemp and cannabis are often used interchangeably, there is a difference. Hemp is defined as a subspecies of the Cannabis sativa L. plant and contains less than 0.3% Tetrahydrocannabinol (THC), so CBD derived from hemp cannot get you "high". THC is the psychoactive chemical in cannabis that is psychogenic, promoting a high or euphoric feeling. The other main subspecies of the Cannabis sativa L. plant is more commonly known as marijuana. The difference is that marijuana contains THC levels greater than 0.3% and is therefore more likely to produce the psychogenic high.

Industrial (or agricultural) hemp is a subspecies strain of the Cannabis sativa plant that has been cultivated worldwide for over 10,000 years because of its vast amount of uses. As explained in chapter 1 of this book, the plant can be refined into a variety of commercial items such as rope, clothing, textiles, insulation, and biofuel. Industrial hemp is grown outdoors, similar to other commodities such as corn or soybeans, and is a very robust plant that can be grown organically without herbicides or pesticides. To legally comply as industrial hemp, the plant must contain no more than 0.3% THC per dry weight. The level of THC in hemp is at least 33 times less than the least potent marijuana strains, so it is nearly impossible for a hemp user to get "high."

Marijuana is the other main subspecies of the cannabis plant that is most frequently harvested for its euphoric, psychoactive properties, which are responsible for making users feel high or stoned. The fibers and stalks of marijuana are not used commercially. Instead, the marijuana plant is cultivated specifically for its flowers, which contain the highest levels of THC in the plant. Physically, marijuana plants typically are bushier and plant strains are selected with a high number of flower, or buds, per plant. Through selective breeding, varieties or strains of marijuana can contain THC concentrations as high as 40% of the dry weight of the plant. Logically, marijuana is naturally lower in CBD than THC.

Molecular-level

Cyclic ring

Hydroxyl group

Tetrahydrocannabinol (THC)

Cannabidiol (CBD)

(The structural formulas of Tetrahydrocannabinol (THC) and Cannabidiol (CBD)) (Source)

At the molecular level, CBD and THC are considered structural isomers which means they share the same chemical composition, but they have different atomic arrangements. The two compounds share a molecular formula of C21H30O2 and molecular weights of 314.5 g/mol.

According to Medical Marijuana, Inc., "The atomic arrangements of the two cannabinoids differ only slightly. Both CBD and THC are considered cyclic compounds, which means one or more series of atoms in the compounds are connected to form a ring. CBD comes with an open ring with a hydroxyl and alkene group, while THC supports a closed ring with an ester group.

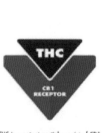
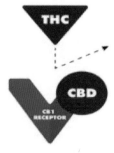

THC is a potent partial agonist of CB1

CBD is a negative allosteric modulator of CB1

Figure 3. Left: THC is a potent partial agonist of CB1. It is this stimulation which leads to the major psychotropic effects of cannabis consumption. Right: CBD is a negative allosteric modulator of CB1 so it changes the shape of the CB1 receptor weakening its ability bind to THC.

(The physiological effects of THC vs CBD) (Source)

28

It's these slight differences in how the atoms of THC and CBD are arranged that have a dramatic effect on how the two cannabinoids interact with the endocannabinoid system's receptors." (Source)

Big Pharma, the Opioid Crisis, and the Revival of Holistic Medicine and Hemp

The Evolution of Big Pharma

In contradiction to the staunch vilification of hemp, the late 1800s and a majority of the 1900s saw a massive revolution in therapeutics. New medicines were being discovered for various ailments by the decade. Opium, Heroin, aspirin, morphine, cocaine, and more, were widely used and purchased as over-the-counter medicines. Along with these new and highly addictive drugs, the U.S. experienced an increase in the misuse

BIG PHARMA NUMBERS

- $329.2 billion - the total amount spent on drugs in 2013

- 12% - the rise in perscription drug cost In the United States every year

- $980 billion - The worldwide pharmaceutical market revenue in 2013

- $1 trillion - The global market for pharmaceuticals topped sales in 2014.

- 1,100+ - The number of paid lobbyists, giving the industry powerful leverage on Capitol Hill.

- $2.9 billion - How much Big Pharma spent on lobbying expenses from 1998-2014.

- $15 million - The amount big pharma doled out more in campaign contributions from 2013-2014.

- 2 - The number of countries in the world whose governments allow prescription drugs to be advertised on TV, the United States is one of them.

and abuse of them. Though a multitude of acts and laws were put into place to subdue the rate of addiction and misuse, new medicines kept popping up and the country began to see more of a divide in terms of beliefs about drugs, even those that were deemed prescriptive.

Although the principles and knowledge of holistic medicine had been around longer than any other medicinal practice, it lost humans' favor once medicines were created. While holistic focused on the health of the whole person — mind, body, spirit, and emotions — and worked from a proactive principle, medicine was thought to be the solution to everything. It reactively treated symptoms and conditions, and for one reason or another, those principles stuck, especially in Western Medicinal practices hundreds of years later.

While there is much (as in we would need to write another dozen books) to be said about the evolution of what has come to be known as Big Pharma, a basic summary should suffice for our purposes. Big Pharma is the nickname given to the world's pharmaceutical industry which includes the trade group Pharmaceutical Research and Manufacturers of America (PhRMA). It is made up of companies that manufacture medical devices, medical supplies, prescription drugs, and more. It has grown to be one of the most powerful industries in the world with global revenues reaching over $1.05 trillion. The U.S. is by far and away the one country where pharmaceutical companies, like Johnson & Johnson, Pfizer, Merck, and others, have gained more power than almost any other industry. The profiteering of the pharmaceutical industry has been growing for over a century with no end in sight. As Gerald Posner notes in his book Pharma: Greed, Lies, and the Poisoning of America, "The highly addictive nature of their products coupled with no government oversight and regulation, was good for sales." Big Pharma was and continues to always be one step ahead of regulation, which has led us to where we are now.

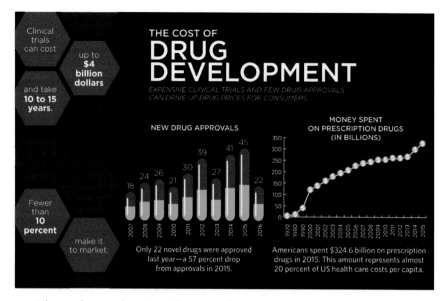

The reality is that Big Pharma often seems to prioritize profits over patients. Drug companies constantly push medical, ethical, and legal boundaries, and the public's reliance on medications as a reactive solution to their ailments has created a perfect storm in which too many of us are drowning.

The Recent Opioid Crisis

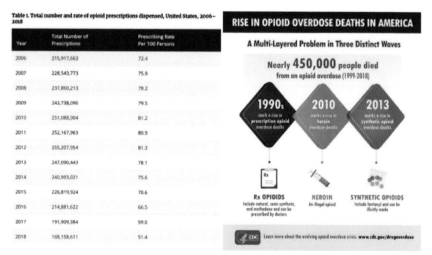

https://www.cdc.gov/drugoverdose/maps/rxrate-maps.html

According to reports from the Centers for Disease Control and Prevention, better known as the CDC, "Opioids were involved in nearly 47,000 deaths in 2018, which is nearly six times the number of opioid-involved overdose deaths in 1999." By the time the U.S. Department of Health and Human Services (HHS) declared it as a public health emergency in 2017, many Americans were puzzled by how we even got so deep without us noticing. Again, while there is a lot more to this issue as a whole, in short, studies and research seem to all lead back to one glaring catalyst. In the late 90s, pharmaceutical companies who were eager to get their medications on the market assured the medical community that opioid pain relievers were not addicting. When healthcare providers saw the effectiveness of the opioids, they increased the number of prescriptions being written which led to a sudden surge of misuse. Unfortunately, the addictive characteristics of opioids took over faster than our knowledge and response to it. For three decades, waves of opioid overdoses (throughout the 90s, in 2010 and again in 2013) led to the CDC rapidly implementing methods to combat the rising epidemic. Their main goals focused on monitoring trends, advancing research, building state, local and tribal capacity, supporting providers, healthcare systems and payers, partnering with public safety officials and community organizations, and increasing public awareness.

The opioid epidemic is far from over and has already taken lives of 450,000 people between 1999-2018[7]. The staggering statistics about opioid-related deaths, not to mention other highly-addictive prescription drugs, has led people to search for safer options to treat their chronic pain. The overlapping relationship between the rise of prescription drugs and the return of hemp products proves that people are beginning to open their eyes and change their minds and opinions about how to care for and treat their bodies.

---

7   https://www.cdc.gov/drugoverdose/epidemic/index.html

The Revival of Holistic/Alternative Medicine and Hemp

As the U.S. saw a rise in medicine's correlation with drug abuse, in the late 1900s, many Americans turned to more holistic or alternative medicine in hopes of achieving optimal health without the use of addicting and chemical-filled drugs. As Jennie Rothenberg Gritz reports, "Enough Americans had similar interests that, in the early 1990s, Congress established an Office of Alternative Medicine within the National Institutes of Health. Seven years later, that office expanded into the National Center for Complementary and Alternative Medicine (NCCAM), with a $50 million budget dedicated to studying just about every treatment that didn't involve pharmaceuticals or surgery—traditional systems like Ayurveda and acupuncture along with more esoteric things like homeopathy and energy healing" (The Atlantic).

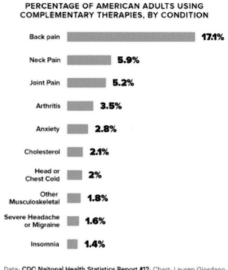

PERCENTAGE OF AMERICAN ADULTS USING COMPLEMENTARY THERAPIES, BY CONDITION

Condition	Percentage
Back pain	17.1%
Neck Pain	5.9%
Joint Pain	5.2%
Arthritis	3.5%
Anxiety	2.8%
Cholesterol	2.1%
Head or Chest Cold	2%
Other Musculoskeletal	1.8%
Severe Headache or Migraine	1.6%
Insomnia	1.4%

Data: CDC Naitonal Health Statistics Report #12; Chart: Lauren Giordano / The Atlantic

According to a 2011 report from the Institute of Medicine, about 100 million American adults suffer from chronic pain—that means about 40 percent of all people over 18. Bringing them relief costs about $560 to $635 billion in incremental healthcare and lost productivity, making pain a more expensive problem than heart disease, cancer, or diabetes.

In the past two decades, thanks to the turn to this newfound desire to embrace more naturalistic lifestyles, hemp is likewise experiencing a revival.

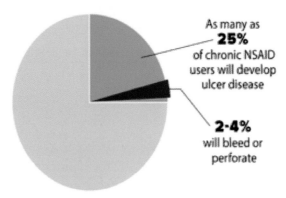

EFFECTS OF CHRONIC NSAID USE
AMONG AMERICANS

As many as
25%
of chronic NSAID
users will develop
ulcer disease

2-4%
will bleed or
perforate

Drugs like ibuprofen and aspirin reduce pain and swelling, but they can also cause serious gastrointestinal complications over time. (Data: The American College of Gastroenterology. Chart: Lauren Giordano / The Atlantic)

It took quite a long time for hemp to make its way back into the (albeit tentative) good graces of the general population, but its reinvigorated popularity has growth-projections of USD 4.6 billion in 2019 to USD 26.6 billion by 2025.[8]

The medical benefits of industrial hemp were highlighted by the 2013 development of a specific high cannabidiol (CBD)/low D9-tetrahydrocannabinol (THC) cannabis strain which helped treat Charlotte Figi, a child who suffered from frequent and severe epileptic seizures not controllable with existing pharmaceuticals.[9] The reports of this "miracle elixir" started the exploration of using hemp extracts to alleviate various ailments. Prior to 2014, industrial hemp was illegal to grow in the United States and extracts were considered controlled substances. However, with growing interest and research, the 2014 Farm Act allowed for pilot studies and research of the hemp plant. Shortly thereafter, the 2018 Agriculture Improvement Act,

---

[8] https://www.prnewswire.com/news-releases/global-industrial-hemp-market-overview--forecast-2019-to-2025-focus-on-hemp-seed-hemp-seed-oil-hemp-fiber-and-cbd-hemp-oil-300879995.html

[9] https://www.cnn.com/2013/08/07/health/charlotte-child-medical-marijuana/index.html
https://www.youtube.com/watch?v=1C6sRkah0mQ

widely known as the Farm Bill, legalized the growth of hemp and hemp extracts at the federal level. More on that in the next chapter.

Because of hemp's many healing properties and ability to be used as both a proactive and reactive therapeutic, CBD can optimize your health and wellness. Later chapters go into much more depth about how and why CBD works in the body, the short explanation is that CBD works remarkably well with our Endocannabinoid System. This system — made up of endocannabinoids, receptors and enzymes — has the ability to regulate the body's internal balance, and simply put, CBD makes for an invaluable player on the endocannabinoid team. Because the endocannabinoid system works in our central nervous system and immune system, when CBD is added as a therapeutic, it can impact and positively effect a wide array of ailments that humans experience on a daily basis.

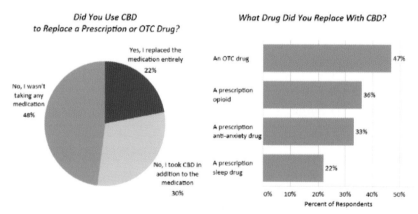

Survey: Consumers Replace Prescription & Over-the-Counter Drugs With CBD

Though in-depth studies about both the Endocannabinoid System and hemp-derived therapeutics are still in their infancy, when considering Big Pharma's corruption and the growing movement toward holistic wellness, CBD is slotted to be a key player in our shifting medicinal practices.

Disruption of Healthcare: the case for CBD

As mentioned in a previous chapter, the medical benefits of industrial hemp were highlighted by the development of a specific high cannabidiol (CBD)/ low D9-tetrahydrocannabinol (THC), the psychogenic component to cannabis) strain to help treat Charlotte Figi, a child who suffered from frequent and severe epileptic seizures that were not controllable with existing pharmaceuticals.

In business theory, a **disruptive innovation** is an innovation that creates a new market and value network and eventually disrupts an existing market and value network, displacing established market-leading firms, products, and alliances. The term was defined and first analyzed by the American scholar Clayton M. Christensen and his collaborators beginning in 1995 and has been called the most influential business idea of the early 21st century.

Not all innovations are disruptive, even if they are revolutionary. For example, the first autos in the late 19th century were not a disruptive innovation, because early automobiles were expensive luxury items that did not disrupt the market for horse drawn vehicles. The market for transportation essentially remained intact until the debut of the lower-priced Model T in 1908. The *mass-produced* automobile was a disruptive innovation, because it changed the transportation market, whereas the first thirty years of automobiles did not.

Disruptive innovations tend to be produced by outsiders in start-ups, rather than existing market-leading companies like pharmaceutical companies. The business environment of market leaders does not allow them to pursue disruptive innovations when they first arise, because they are not profitable enough at first and because their development can take scarce resources away from sustaining innovations (which are needed to compete against current competition). Small teams are more likely to create disruptive innovations than large teams. A disruptive process can take longer to develop than by the conventional approach and the risk associated to it is higher than the other more incremental or evolutionary forms of innovations, but once it is deployed in the market, it achieves a much faster penetration and higher degree of impact on the established markets. (Source Wikipedia)

Are Cannabinoids a disruptive innovation?

The reports of this "miracle elixir" started the exploration of using hemp extracts to alleviate various ailments. Today, hemp extracts have been anecdotally reported to treat as many as 100 different health conditions ranging from anti-infective to treating tumors. Although some of these health claims may not be valid, early clinical studies demonstrate that hemp extracts may effectively treat a variety of inflammatory conditions, provide a pain relief alternative, alleviate anxiety, and increase sleep quality.

Medicinal Values (human and animals)

No, CBD will not miraculously cure cancer, but there is <u>some evidence</u> that it might be a helpful supplement with symptoms.

Other CBD Applications

There are FDA approved medications that have CBD as one of the main active ingredients that are not Epidiolex or based around epilepsy at all. Most of them are for helping fight the nausea that is a common side effect of cancer treatments. Another one is called Sativex. That one is made to help combat the spastic pain that comes along with multiple sclerosis.

As you can see, the Schedule V designation on Epidiolex is nothing more than a way of saying that it is considered to be safe overall by both the FDA and the DEA. There is still more research that needs to be done on CBD and CBD based medications. As time goes on it will be interesting to see what medications are approved by the FDA and the DEA.

How CBD Works in the Body: Physiology

The human body is significantly more nuanced and complex than most people think. Many discoveries amaze even the most prolific of scientists.

One recurring theme in many of these discoveries is that there are systems and interactions within the human body that are highly specialized yet play a critical role in our well-being. For example, there might be a receptor that responds only to a specific molecule, but that molecule might be the difference between feeling well and having poor health.

In 1988, researchers expounded more on the endocannabinoid system, and it is the perfect example of a highly valuable set of interactions that had previously gone undetected because it was so nuanced. While research is still emerging, there is evidence that endocannabinoids are involved in everything from inflammation to anxiety to sleep. There is even evidence to suggest that endocannabinoids are involved in brain and heart health. The best part is that CBD, which is a cannabinoid, works with this system and helps unlock its full potential.

To understand this system better and see how it can help you, we need to first look at how the system functions.

Endocannabinoids: A Critical Component of Natural Health

The prefix "endo" is a Greek term that means "within." An endocannabinoid system, therefore, is a set of biochemicals that our body generates and receptors that function when the biochemicals bind.

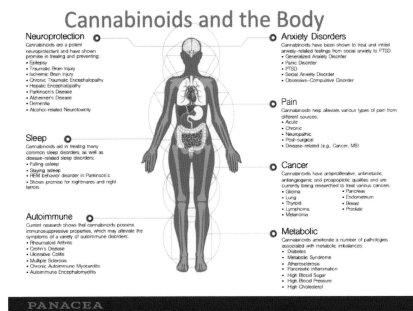

Cannabinoids and the Body

Neuroprotection
Cannabinoids are a potent neuroprotectant and have shown promise in treating and preventing:
- Epilepsy
- Traumatic Brain Injury
- Ischemic Brain Injury
- Chronic Traumatic Encephalopathy
- Hepatic Encephalopathy
- Parkinson's Disease
- Alzheimer's Disease
- Dementia
- Alcohol-related Neurotoxicity

Sleep
Cannabinoids aid in treating many common sleep disorders, as well as disease-related sleep disorders:
- Falling asleep
- Staying asleep
- REM behavior disorder in Parkinson's
- Shows promise for nightmares and night terrors

Autoimmune
Current research shows that cannabinoids possess immunosuppressive properties, which may alleviate the symptoms of a variety of autoimmune disorders:
- Rheumatoid Arthritis
- Crohn's Disease
- Ulcerative Colitis
- Multiple Sclerosis
- Chronic Autoimmune Myocarditis
- Autoimmune Encephalomyelitis

Anxiety Disorders
Cannabinoids have been shown to treat and inhibit anxiety-related feelings from social anxiety to PTSD:
- Generalized Anxiety Disorder
- Panic Disorder
- PTSD
- Social Anxiety Disorder
- Obsessive–Compulsive Disorder

Pain
Cannabinoids help alleviate various types of pain from different sources:
- Acute
- Chronic
- Neuropathic
- Post-surgical
- Disease-related (e.g. Cancer, MS)

Cancer
Cannabinoids have antiproliferative, antimetastatic, antiangiogenic and proapoptotic qualities and are currently being researched to treat various cancers:
- Glioma
- Lung
- Thyroid
- Lymphoma
- Melanoma
- Pancreas
- Endometrium
- Breast
- Prostate

Metabolic
Cannabinoids ameliorate a number of pathologies associated with metabolic imbalances:
- Diabetes
- Metabolic Syndrome
- Atherosclerosis
- Pancreatic inflammation
- High Blood Sugar
- High Blood Pressure
- High Cholesterol

Many of the body's processes work on the principle of receptors and chemicals that bind to those receptors, eliciting some response. A perfect example of this is serotonin in the brain. Serotonin binds to receptors in the brain to create feelings of happiness. Having too little serotonin can induce feelings of anxiety and depression. Serotonin does more for your body than merely regulate mood, but within the brain, some receptors look for this chemical and bind to it.

The endocannabinoid system is similar. There are cannabinoids that the body produces naturally, and there are receptors throughout our body that detect for them. When these endocannabinoids bind with these receptors, it signals to our bodies to do a specific action. Remarkably, these receptors bind not just with the cannabinoids that our body produces, but also with cannabinoids found in the cannabis plant. The two major cannabinoids, THC and CBD, both bind with these receptors, but in very different ways.

There are two types of cannabinoid receptors. Many scientific papers abbreviate them as CB-1 and CB-2.

CB-1 receptors are in the brain primarily, though they are also in reproductive systems and the cerebellum. These receptors are involved in many functions. In particular, they are partly responsible for "movement, sensory learning, analgesia, anxiety, and appetitive behaviors." Within the body, the primary cannabinoids that bind with this receptor are anandamide and 2-Arachidonoylglycerol (2-AG). The brain contains these natural compounds, and they play essential roles in regulating the behaviors listed.

Your immune system and peripheral nervous system contain CB-2 receptors. The brain and your gastrointestinal system also contain these receptors. Like, CB-1, CB-2 also plays a critical role within the human body. Most notably, CB-2 regulates inflammation. Binding with these receptors can moderate the behavior of our immune system, particularly when it becomes overly active. There is also evidence that these receptors have neuroprotective properties. In our bodies, the main endocannabinoid that binds with this receptor is 2-AG, which also interacts with CB-1.

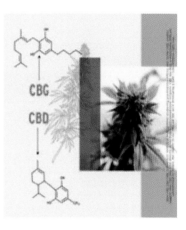

Both receptors, and the chemical compounds that couple with them, work to achieve homeostasis within our bodies. They keep our bodily processes, like eating and immune response to infection, relatively stable so our bodies can function in good health. Indeed, without the endocannabinoid system, we might not even be able to work correctly! That is likely one of the biggest reasons why most mammals have this system.

THC And CBD: Cannabinoids That Also Bind

As cannabinoids, both THC and CBD also bind to CB-1 and CB-2 receptors, but the way they do so is very different. THC binds to CB-1 receptors primarily and partially binds to CB-2. Recall that CB-1 is responsible for things like movement and appetitive behaviors. When someone smokes Marijuana, they ingest THC. Our bodies absorb that compound, which makes its way to the CB-1 receptors. When it binds with them, it creates the familiar "high" sensation about which Marijuana users are very familiar. The fact that the CB-1 receptor also regulates appetite explains the infamous "munchies" that Marijuana smokers get.

On the other hand, CBD binds to CB-2 receptors but doesn't attach well to CB-1 ones. That explains why CBD is a well-known immunosuppressant. Under normal circumstances, immune cells release cannabinoids to signal other cells, but also let our bodies know that the fighting of the infection is underway. The cannabinoids make their way to the CB-2 receptors, and our body knows cells are "on-site and working," so to speak.

In some respects, you might think of the CB-2 receptors in immune cells as phoning methods. When there is a fire, someone calls in the emergency. When crews arrive, they also radio in to say that they are there fighting the blaze. Your immune system works similarly. When your body detects an unknown pathogen, it needs to send cells to the site to destroy it. But you don't want the system to become over-active and destroy everything. Instead, the immune system partly uses the CB-2 receptor to say, "Hey, we're here at the scene of infection and are fighting it," so that way your body doesn't need to dispatch too many immune cells.

By taking CBD, we activate these receptors, which, in turn, moderates our immune system. For people with healthy immune system responses, this won't do much. However, for people with overactive immune systems, CBD has the potential to have a significant impact. With diseases of the immune system, such as rheumatoid arthritis, the immune system attacks healthy tissue. These attacks cause the joint to become inflamed and result in pain, swelling, and a whole slew of undesirable complications.

CBD is a natural way to suppress an overactive immune system and help it not attack healthy tissue. In turn, the inflammation won't happen, and the muscle or connective tissue can remain healthy. In rheumatoid arthritis, for example, the immune system continuously destroys the connective tissue, which causes extreme pain and difficulty moving the joint. CBD may help keep the inflammation away and let the joint heal and function like it did before arthritis.

The fact that CBD does not bind well to CB-1 receptors also explains why people do not have a "high" sensation from CBD but do feel some level of happiness and anxiety relief. It's not that CBD does not bind at all to CB-1 receptors; it just does so significantly less than THC. It attaches to these receptors at such a low level that CBD is not psychoactive, and people retain full cognition and mental state after taking CBD.

Intriguingly, CBD can also help to mitigate the effects of THC. When administered together, CBD will bind primarily to CB-2 and a little to the CB-1 receptors. In small doses, CBD may have an "inverse agonist" effect on CB-1 receptors. This term means that it binds to the CB-1 receptor but has the opposite effect of an agonist like THC. Therefore, if CBD binds first, it has the effect of blocking the THC, thereby lessening some of the results that THC can have on people's mental states. Marijuana contains both CBD and THC, so the "high" that people feel while consuming it is reduced in part due to the presence of CBD.

How Does CBD Promote Natural Health?

Part of the success of CBD is that it works with our endocannabinoid system in a complementary way. It is a substance that is natural and that our bodies expect to have in it. We even have receptors that work with these cannabinoids. This natural extract, of course, stands in stark contrast with manufactured medicines which are synthetically produced and oftentimes have undesired side effects. While you should never stop taking your prescribed medication, it also doesn't hurt to look at all-natural solutions about which you can talk with your doctor.

There are a few ways in which CBD promotes natural health. The first way, of course, is by reducing inflammation. As described earlier, CBD's ability to bind with the CB-2 receptor has an immunosuppressive effect. If you have an autoimmune disease, CBD may help you. This includes everything from rheumatoid arthritis to lupus to psoriasis to multiple sclerosis. Of course, you should discuss taking CBD with your doctor for any of these conditions, but there is emerging research that suggests it may be beneficial.

The other way CBD promotes an improved quality of life is through a reduction in anxiety and stress. Recall that CBD has a mild "inverse agonist" effect on CB-1 receptors. The THC compound, which is an agonist, tends to induce anxiety when smoking Marijuana. Counterbalancing that anxiety is CBD, which, when binding to the CB-1 receptors, has an inverse effect.

Of course, if you take CBD and have no other compounds that aggressively bind with the CB-1 receptor, then the CBD will unite with some of them as well and make you feel more relaxed. This reason is why many CBD users report less anxiety and less stress.

That relaxed feeling that CBD users experience has other positive benefits. Feeling less stressed can result in lower blood pressure and has various cardiovascular benefits. Since CBD may have the ability to reduce anxiety and depression, it can help protect against these things. There is also some research to suggest that CBD oil, much like fish oil, is an antioxidant. In effect, this property means that it helps protect your cells from damage. Research has consistently shown that this property helps fish oil protect your heart. CBD oil may have similar features when it comes to your heart.

There is also some evidence to suggest that CBD may have neuroprotective properties. The reason why it may help boost brain health is, again, due to these receptors. In the brain, CB-2 receptors tend to have presynaptic-inhibition. There is some evidence to suggest that this type of inhibition has neuroprotective qualities. Since CBD is good at binding to these endocannabinoid receptors, it then follows that it would help protect and promote brain health.

CBD And the Endocannabinoid System: A Perfect Match

Many CBD and Marijuana users are surprised when they learn that our bodies have specialized systems that work with the compounds in cannabis. We likely didn't evolve these specialized systems because there is a plant. Instead, it just happens that this plant contains compounds that our systems can use in a meaningful and beneficial way.

The endocannabinoid system has two primary receptors, CB-1 and CB-2. Under normal circumstances, there are two compounds within our bodies that bind to these receptors. These substances are anandamide and 2-Arachidonoylglycerol. 2-AG, the latter compound, also links with CB-2. When your body is functioning normally, these two cannabinoids are produced internally and trigger the appropriate responses.

However, when you ingest CBD or THC, these compounds interfere with these systems. THC binds with CB-1 to make you feel anxious, hungry, and give you a "high" sensation. Conversely, CBD binds with CB-2 to help reduce inflammation, anxiety, depression, and potentially help with a whole slew of health issues. While both compounds serve their purpose, CBD is more health-oriented, whereas THC is more pleasure-oriented.

It's worth noting that CBD research is still in its infancy. Remember that researchers only found this entire system within our bodies in 1992. That date makes the investigations less than 30 years old. Also, researchers into the benefits of CBD have had to jump through hoops due to CBD's unfortunate association with Marijuana. As such, the bulk of the research has only occurred within the past decade or so.

The Future of Cannabinoids

More Potential Pathways for Hemp Research

Given the fact that this bill has opened the door for legalized CBD and hemp, restrictions on hemp and CBD research have also been lessened. The 2018 Farm Bill goes even further than merely permitting this research to happen legally – it expressly "provides USDA oversight and funding for hemp research." In other words, we should expect to see researchers all across the US looking into the various ways that industrial hemp can be beneficial. While there is nothing in this directive that targets CBD specifically, given the interest in CBD and its potential health benefits – as well as the FDA who wants to take an official stance on the subject based on science – we will likely see more research into this topic in the future.

A few years ago, the hemp CBD market had barely hit the radar. Nowadays, CBD has spread into other markets, including pharmaceuticals, cosmetics, and even food. Arcview Market Research projects that the collective market for CBD sales in the U.S. will surpass $20 billion by 2024. With this much of an opportunity currently coming from dispensaries, pharmaceuticals, and general retail, a lot of the analysis predicts more of this opportunity will come from general retail stores.

When you consider how much cannabis has become integrated into today's society and the increased information available, it easy to see that the market share for CBD and even THC will skyrocket. While legalization is currently being sought on a federal level, many states have exercised their power and have opened up more opportunities than they initially expected.

With an annual growth rate of forty-nine percent by 2024 across all distribution channels is easy to see how CBD will dominate a good section of the market. Combine this with THC products, will create a total market share of $45 billion for cannabinoids by 2024. With full legalization eventually coming to pass, the market share of CBD will likely increase along with research and development of new brands and products. Support of legalization is growing amongst all political ideologies, and though there will be tight regulation on federal and state levels, neither will prevent the market from growing or even stagnating anytime soon. The nation will sincerely benefit from an improved legal status as a growing audience of people seek healthier and better alternatives for a new lifestyle.

Bioavailability and Delivery Methods

Bioavailability refers to the extent and rate at which the active moiety (drug or metabolite) enters systemic circulation, thereby accessing the site of action. **Bioavailability** of a drug is largely determined by the properties of the dosage form, which depend partly on its design and manufacture.

There are several ways to improve bioavailability in CBD products. For example, Full Spectrum Oil is an oil that consists of the cannabinoids, terpenes, and flavonoids present in the hemp plant. hemp FSO will be high in CBD content, low in THC, but contain other minor cannabinoids. Most plants produce terpenes to deter predators and give unique smells to the plant. For example, conifers express pinene, a terpene that provides the pine scent associated with various trees. Terpenes have health benefits that compliment cannabinoids. Similarly, flavonoids give plant extracts their unique taste, and have additional health benefits. We choose to make many of our products with full-spectrum hemp oil to provide the greatest health benefits possible. In addition, other complimentary ingredients are added to interact with the terpenes and distillate to provide maximum bioavailability.

Panacea Life Sciences F.A.S.T.

Bioavailability

Bioavailability is the amount of the active medication absorbed into the patient's bloodstream. The higher the bioavailability, the higher the potential efficacy.

Bioavailability Comparison of Different Routes of Administration

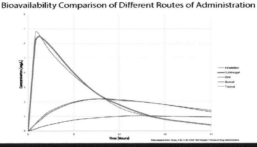

Broad Spectrum Oil is an oil that consists of the cannabinoids, terpenes, and flavonoids present in the hemp plant less the THC. Hemp BSO will be high in CBD content, non-detectable THC, but contain other minor cannabinoids. Most plants produce terpenes to deter predators and give unique smells to the plant. For example, conifers express pinene, a terpene that provides the pine scent associated with various trees. Terpenes have health benefits that compliment cannabinoids. Similarly, flavonoids give plant extracts their unique taste, and have additional health benefits. We choose to make many of our products with full-spectrum hemp oil to provide the greatest health benefits possible.

Delivery Methods

Sublinguals

Sublingual refers to a product being absorbed under your tongue.

Our Fast Acting Sublingual Tablets, or F.A.S.T. Tablets, are unique to Panacea Life Sciences and are designed to offer the highest bioavailability on the market. The tablets dissolve under your tongue in seconds and are more reliable than tinctures, as each tablet delivers a targeted, consistent dose of

CBD in every tablet. Tinctures are hard to judge and the CBD can fluctuate from drop to drop.

Ingestibles

These products and edibles are absorbed in the digestive tract. These are great for time released products and oils that are not particularly palatable (don't taste good). Our DAILY line of soft gels are our preferred application in this category. They are time released to offer higher bioavailability and long lasting effects for our FULL SPECTRUM and other oil based formulations. Compare this to other ingestibles that typically see about 10-20% absorption and can lead to waste and, most importantly, ineffective results.

Topicals

Topicals are any products that are applied to the skin. Here, the ingredients are absorbed through the pores and cell walls on your skin and, in the case of our SOOTHE products, act to relieve pain and inflammation locally. Topicals are great for spot treating sore joints, muscles, and other injuries that can be reached through the skin. Topicals can also be restorative, like our Transform Face Crème, which is a great compliment to therapeutic massage and/ or combined with other products for a "full body" treatment.

There are a few reasons why people use CBD topicals. The main ones are to combat inflammation and as a boost to skin health. While the research on what CBD can do to benefit those things is still preliminary, it is promising.

Inflammation is something that can cause a lot of problems, for a lot of people. It can lead to discomfort and even pain. So, dealing with it can be difficult. One study published in 2013 found that CBD helps act as an anti-inflammatory in mice. This is just one study of many out there looking at the anti-inflammatory effects of CBD. Using topicals for this purpose may be more effective as the topicals tend to keep their effects in the area that you apply them. That means that it will be more concentrated in places where you are feeling the most inflammation.

Skincare is important for everyone. If you are struggling with acne, many products can be discouraging as they can mix with the oils on your skin and exacerbate the issue. CBD may be able to help with this. As this Healthline article lays out, CBD may help reduce the body's production of sebum, the oil that while protecting our skin, can also clog up our pores. This means that your odds of experiencing breakout may drop when using CBD.

If you are taking medications for either of these issues, be sure to talk to your doctor before stopping or changing the way you take your medications.

Tinctures (oils)

To understand what CBD oil is, we must first understand how it is made. This CBD is extracted from the Cannabis plant. Because CBD has such a high concentration, the hemp oil is diluted by using carrier oils. There are many different types of carrier oils including coconut, Aragon, avocado, grape seed, and the most popular type found in CBD oil, hemp seed oil. hemp seed oil alone does not carry CBD so, purchasing hemp seed oil does not provide the potential benefits that CBD does. Carrier oils assist the CBD oil for ingestion and also topical use. Here at Panacea Life Sciences, we produce our own CBD oil. This CBD oil contains palm oil and is our most popular product. Our CBD oil contains 99% CBD oil and comes in natural, mixed berry and vanilla flavors. The typical administration of CBD oil is to place an amount under a person's tongue. The sublingual membrane in your mouth allow the CBD to reach the bloodstream very quickly.

Tinctures are simply concentrated extracts. There are several ways to extract CBD into a tincture. This article explains the three main ways to extract CBD. They include carbon dioxide, hydrocarbon/natural solvents, and steam distillation.

1. **Steam Distillation:** During this process, the steam removes the CBD oil from the plant. The plant that the processor wants to extract from is placed in a container that is separate from a boiler full of water. The Cannabis plant is then placed above the boiler and as the steam

from the water rises, it separates the hemp oil containing CBD from the plant. The fumes from the plant are then trapped in a tube and then added to water or oil. After this is condensed, the oil is extracted from the water (if used) to create an oil.

2. **Solvent Extraction (Hydrocarbons and Natural Solvents):** This process is similar to the steam distillation extraction method. Rather than using an oil or water to place the extracted CBD in a solvent is used. The solvent of choice is combined with the CBD oil, then the solvent is extracted and producing CBD hemp oil. The type of solvent used varies. The two commonly used are natural solvents and hydrocarbons solvents. This type of extraction is the least popular because it may leave unwanted items behind after the solvent has been extracted. These elements could include butane, propane, or naphtha when hydrocarbon extraction is used.

3. **Carbon Dioxide Extraction:** this type of extraction, known as supercritical fluid extraction (SFE), uses both carbon dioxide liquid and gas properties. This type of extraction is also known as Supercritical Fluid Extraction or SFE. To start this extraction, hemp is placed into a chamber that is then filled with liquid carbon dioxide under pressure. The hemp-CO2 liquid is then pumped into an expansion chamber where the CO2 is allowed to sublimate into gas which is recaptured for the next round of extraction. The remaining liquid is a beautiful, caramel-colored hemp oil free of any solvents.

The taste of a CBD tincture varies from tincture to tincture. The general taste of CBD oil is often described as nut-like, earthy, or grassy. These tinctures can be used under the tongue, and that is when the taste is generally quite strong. Some users enjoy the taste of the tincture, and others do not. There are other ways to take CBD oil. But, if you want the full effects of the tincture oil, you can place it in various things for ingestion. If you want to use the oil, consider swallowing the tincture with yogurt or adding it to your morning smoothie. Adding the CBD tincture to sweet food items may mask the earthy flavors of the CBD oil while still allowing you to receive the full benefits. However, there are still multiple different ways to get CBD daily that are not tinctures.

How dosing works

The definition of dosage or dose is "the quantity of an active agent (substance or radiation) taken in or absorbed at any one time." It is likely you've heard this term used when taking most types of medication. To be clear, CBD is not a medication, but does have amounts of "active agents" and uses the measurement system of mg (milligrams) that are to be administered.

There is no one set amount of CBD that is right for people of a particular age or weight. Everyone reacts to the cannabinoid a little bit differently, and while weight and age can play a part, they are not the only factors to consider. So, when starting CBD for the first time, you may have to do some experimentation.

Before we can talk about how to find the right amount of CBD, we need to talk about what to avoid while taking the cannabinoid. CBD is considered to be safe overall. However, it does have some negative side effects. They are normally associated with taking too much CBD and consist of things like nausea and dizziness. While not life threatening, those side effects are still not fun, and you should do your best to avoid them. Of course, the way to do that is by finding the right amount of CBD for you.

The best way to go about starting to take CBD is by keeping the initial amount as low as you can. After taking that, wait a little while and see how it sits with you. If after an hour or so you do not notice any negative side effects, but you also are not seeing the effects that you are looking for, then you can try taking some more. It is important to go about this carefully. Do not just take CBD until you experience negative side effects. Whatever is the smallest amount that does not give you any negative side effects but does give you the positive effect you are looking for, then that is amount for you.

You should also note that CBD does not mix well with all medication. It causes some medications to have a lessened effect and others to stop working entirely. If you are taking medications and want to start using CBD, be sure to discuss it with your healthcare provider first. They should know whether or not your medications will safely mix with CBD.

It is also important to know that most CBD products are intended for those who are 18 or older. Keep CBD products out of reach of children. Especially products, like edibles, that do not look very different from their non-CBD equivalents.

The examples of research that has been done on CBD in this article are just that, examples. This article only went over a couple of the areas that researchers have been looking into, so there is even more to know. There is so much research that has been done on the cannabinoid. There is even more yet to come. As the years pass, we will likely learn more about what potential benefits the cannabinoid may hold for us.

Our products are unique and they are extremely safe. Because these products have a very high safety ratio (over 1000 fold), which is the ratio of concentrations where health benefits are achieved versus adverse events, consumers can explore the right concentration of Panacea products to take for their specific health goal. Our preclinical studies indicate that to maintain joint health, function, and flexibility, a dose ranging from 0.4 mg/kg/day to 2 mg/kg/day is suggested. Note that a person's body weight and degree of discomfort will influence the amount of material needed to be taken to experience positive effects. For example, our Cherry Bomb CBD Gummies have 20mg of CBD in each piece and our daily softgels are available in 10mg, 25mg, and 50mg tablets.

We suggest two soft gels per day, one in the morning and one in the evening. The consumer should experiment and decide what works for them and their condition. Panacea manufactures a low, medium, and high strength formula to help consumers tailor the CBD dosage needed for their specific situation. The amount of CBD that should be administered varies from person to person. Like most things that are new, we also suggest starting with a low amount of CBD. Eventually, your body will become more accustomed to the CBD and the amount one takes may differ until they find the perfect dose. It is important to speak with a physician before taking CBD, as it may have effects on medications that are taken alongside it. Again, starting low and increasing the amount will help you figure out what dose is right for you. This way the effects will not vary from time to time and you will get all the potential benefits.

Can you overdose on CBD?

Despite the fact that CBD is generally considered safe and non-addictive, you may wonder about the potential for overdose. After all, there are many drugs out there that don't seem dangerous but carry pretty stern warnings about toxicity levels.

Fortunately, there have been no documented cases of anyone overdosing on CBD thus far. Because CBD effects are generally mild and therapeutic rather than intoxicating, you are not going to become "too high" like you might with some other drugs.

You cannot lethally overdose on CBD, but it is still possible to have too much (just like with any other substance). Taking pure CBD in large amounts won't kill you, but it might lead to drowsiness, diarrhea and dizziness. To avoid this, simply follow the directions on your CBD product. Most studies show that humans can handle up to 1500 milligrams of CBD per day without any issues.

Luckily, there doesn't seem to be any amount of CBD that can be considered dangerous for human consumption – just levels that may make for some mild discomfort. Because our body naturally produces cannabidiol, we are already used to it and can use it for therapeutic purposes. The most likely scenario if you have more CBD than you are used to is that you will become more tired than usual. For some people, this may be a desired effect.

The most important thing is to start slowly with your CBD consumption to see how much is right for you. If you don't notice any effects right away, you can slowly add more to your routine and you don't have to worry about becoming ill or overdosing.

Panacea Life Sciences: What Makes Us Unique

The Panacea Story

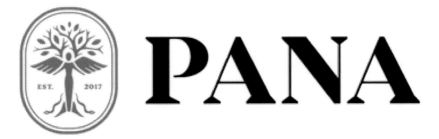

When her 78-year-old mother suffered a fractured pelvis, Leslie Buttorff's devotion to helping her mother find pain-relief quickly led to the creation of Panacea Life Sciences. The idea became apparent when she was beta testing Quintel-MC, Inc.'s ERPCannabis software – an enterprise resource planning tool for marijuana companies that were struggling to run back-office operations and track seed-to-sale transactions. As Buttorff's knowledge grew, she geared her focus toward CBD and hemp. After through various acquisitions and mergers in late 2017, she named her company after the Greek goddess of healing and remedies, Panacea. Leslie's mother is now 82 years old, and with the relief from daily CBD F.A.S.T. tablets, she is able to take Zumba classes and lead her normal life. Looking back, she credits her daughter's dedication to her eagerness in "helping people and pets feel better every day by delivering the highest-quality CBD products on the market".

In 2018, the company focused on extraction and softgel and tablet production in a small demonstration laboratory in Louisville, Colorado. Given the considerable number of sales the company acquired, it was critical to move to a larger location, so in December 2018, a 51,000 sq. ft building was purchased in the Coors Tech Center in Golden, Colorado. The facility was previously used by the EPA; thus, it was already designed for laboratory use and dangerous materials. The company soon expanded all its testing, extraction and production capabilities.

The year 2019 was another productive year that yielded substantial growth thanks in large part to the acquisition of Needle Rock Hemp Farms in October. This beautiful piece of property is on the western slope of Colorado and is surrounded by Rocky Mountain springs. The property includes 240 acres and has the capacity to supply all the hemp required for Panacea's products. Shortly after, in December 2019, Panacea and Twenty Second Century (NYSE XXII) (a biomedical and cannabinoid research company) completed a deal where Panacea would have access to capital and XXII's proprietary research for various THC-free hemp strains. Finally, to round out the successful year, Buttorff — who has tight ties with her alma mater, Colorado State University — donated $1.5 million to build a center for cannabinoid research. Panacea and CSU have since teamed up with the intention to discover new cannabinoids and testing techniques. The lab was scheduled to open in April 2020 but was delayed due to COVID-19.

Much like years prior, 2020 started off as exciting year for additional CBD growth but unfortunately was somewhat curtailed by the COVID-19 virus. The company quickly pivoted some of its resources to making hand sanitizers. The remainder of 2020 will be spent on refining our processes and building modifications to complete our Current Goods Manufacturing Processes (cGMP) and ISO9001 audit recommendations, as well as expanding our product lines with our new branding initiative. The goal for 2021 is to expand our CBD and CBG cosmetic line and introduce our line of CBG products.

What's in a name?

The original design for the logo reflected the original mission: to bring medical quality hemp oil to patients in need. The symbolic elements of the logo included the Panacea goddess in the center, which is represented entwined with a Caduceus, a symbol representing modern medicine in the United

Caduceus

An ancient Greek or Roman herald's wand, typically one with two serpents twined around it, carried by the messenger god Hermes or Mercury.

States. The medical symbol is laid over a plant motif representing life as well as our commitment to providing natural plant extracts.

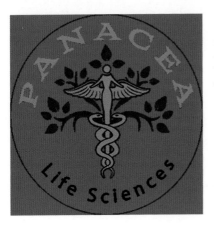

In Greek Mythology, Panacea is the goddess of universal remedy. Panacea was said to have a potion with which she helped the sick. This brought about the concept of the panacea in medicine.

The tree symbolizes the "breath of life" and healing aspects. We believe these three symbols reflect the potential of natural oils derived from the hemp plant to provide relief for several human conditions or as a panacea.

As Panacea Life Sciences has grown as a company, so too have our branding and mission statement. This growth is illustrated by our new brand standards on all levels.

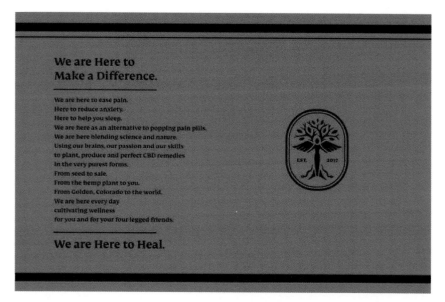

The biggest change is an outcome of our immense growth into several different channels in the hemp industry. Since the start of Panacea Life Sciences, we have come to see the value in cultivating everyday wellness, and our new customer-facing products now boast the name "Pana" which encompasses six ancillary product lines. Stemming from the Greek language, Pan refers to "all". By using PANA as our name, we speak to the all-natural ingredients and holistic healing that PANA offers.

The newer goddess logomark is the visual representation of the brand. Inspired by Panacea, the Greek goddess of healing, the PANA mark represents the three brand equities of Nature, Nurture and Science, while the logotype captures our scientific yet nurturing essence.

Why we're different

Vertically Integrated

Growing and processing the hemp plant presents unique concerns that require proper growing conditions to ensure the resulting plant extracts are free from contaminants. Furthermore, careful attention to extraction procedures that may introduce additional contaminants into the oil, and therefore

60

must be removed, makes the manufacturing process difficult and meticulous. These issues together have resulted in an industry-wide lack of quality control, leading to over 50% of today's commercialized products to fail potency and purity quality requirements that are standard for other product categories. Quality issues are the main reasons why retailers must perform due diligence in choosing a manufacturer and CBD product line. One strategy is hemp manufacturers are utilizing to increase quality of products is to become vertically integrated, meaning the company controls the entire process from growing the hemp, extraction, production of CBD-oil, and manufacturing finished products, recently coined as the phrase "seed to sale".

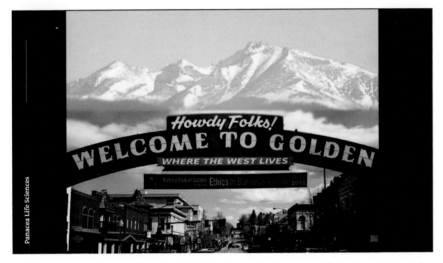

Panacea Life Sciences

Panacea is focused on creating high quality, organic hemp and cannabidiol (CBD) products for those seeking to lead a healthier lifestyle. Our focus on creating plant-based health and wellness products to deliver top quality products for specific needs for humans and pets. To achieve our mission, we have created a completely vertically integrated company that controls our supply chain and manufacturing process from seed to sale. We grow the highest quality CBD biomass in Colorado to input to our products and use the most rigorous SOPs for our stringent GMP-level extraction and manufacturing processes. Simply stated, we develop products to improve the lives of our consumers through cannabinoid-based products that work.

By owning the hemp farm, CBD manufacturers are not only able to produce CBD oils with elevated minor cannabinoids and terpenes but can also ensure the plants are free from contaminants.

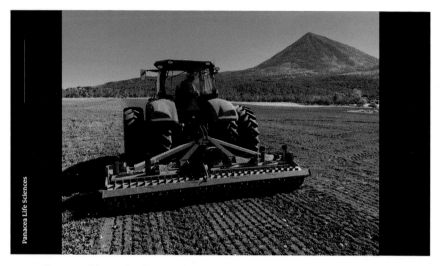

Where and how the hemp plant is grown is especially important as hemp is a hyper-accumulator of contaminants in the soil. In recent Hemp News, they stated that Delta County CO is the number 1 place in the work to grow hemp due to many favorable characteristics. Any heavy metals or organic contaminants in the soil will be absorbed by the roots of the hemp plant and stored in the leaves and flowers used to make CBD oil. Because hemp has the complex characteristics of a deep tap root that can penetrate the soil up to 8 feet, a rapid growth cycle of 12 weeks, and very efficiently absorbs pollutants in the soil, hemp is often used for phytoremediation, or restoring, of contaminated fields. In fact, farmers in Italy have successfully cleansed dioxin contaminated fields, and the University of Virginia has performed studies on how hemp can be used to clean up contamination from coal processing. The hemp plant has even been used to help remediate radioactive contamination from the 1986 Chernobyl nuclear reactor disaster. For these reasons, among others, vertically integrated hemp companies will ensure their hemp crops are organically compliant to minimize crop contamination, and most companies will work towards organic certification of their growing operation which first became available to the hemp industry late last year (2019).

The Four Key Takeaways About Panacea Life Sciences

1. Our objective is to address inconsistencies in dosing by providing consumers with extremely consistent, high quality, pharmaceutical grade products. We grow carefully curated strains, infuse, formulate, produce, and package products on site to strictly control the production process.

2. Our products contain our organically grown hemp grown in Delta County, CO. Our hemp is grown with no pesticides or fertilizers. The plants are hand-picked for our extraction process.

3. Once the oil is extracted from the hemp plant, we formulate the resulting oil into unique formulations that provide the highest bioavailability compared to other companies.

4. All of our products are manufactured in the USA using Good Manufacturing Practice (GMP) which ensures that Panacea products will consistently contain the needed hemp oil in every dose for maximal effects.

The seed to sale process

Panacea Life Sciences, Inc. acquired Needle Rock Farms (NRF) located on the western slope of Colorado in November 2019. Needle Rock Farms had been growing hemp for the past five years. The acquisition included 235 acres of farmland, water rights, farm equipment, barns, greenhouses and irrigation systems, as well as the 2019 hemp grow cycle. The farm is slated to achieve its organic certification in 2020, and further plans include establishing the farm as a production facility and grow two of the most popular strains of hemp. Rocky mountain spring water—which is crystal clear and high in nutrients—is used for the grow. PANA Organic Botanicals at Needle Rock will provide Panacea's hemp for years to come.

The strategy behind the acquisition of the farm was two-fold. First, it was important to control our raw hemp materials and for the hemp farm to be certified, organic hemp farm. With this acquisition we now control the entire value chain for the production of our products. This was an important criterion for many retail stores and others that now require seed to sale tracking. Second, the hemp market is very volatile and it is a very difficult crop to grow, so prices vary widely and overall quality is an issue. Nine out of ten samples we received last year were rejected. By owning the hemp farm, CBD manufacturers are not only able to produce CBD oils with elevated minor cannabinoids and terpenes but can also ensure the plants are free from contaminants.

Here's a look at how Panacea processes our CBD and CBG products from seed to sale.

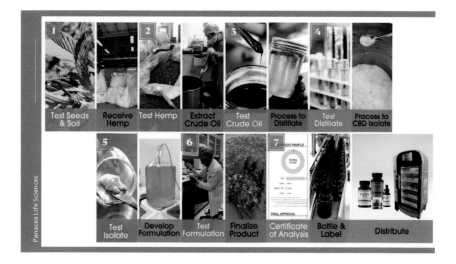

01 Seed to Clones to Plant

We start with selected varieties of hemp seeds and grow our mother plants. Those female plants that are most desirable are then cloned for consistency, and nurtured in a greenhouse, and planted with organic practices into our fields to ensure the highest quality hemp for our products.

02 Flower

When they are mature, the flower is harvested from these premium plants. This is the biomass used for extraction.

03 Decarboxylation

The flower is heated up in a process called decarboxylation to convert the CBDA to CBD and to provide the highest amount of CBD possible.

04 Crude

The decarboxylated biomass is extracted naturally to provide CBD crude oil.

05 Terpenes

By carefully choosing the variety of plants, and isolating these delicate terpenes from our biomass, we are able to provide the most pleasant characteristic aroma in our products.

06 Process To Distillate

Using specialized chemical equipment, the crude oil is distilled. The desired cannabinoids are purified and enriched during this process.

07 Process to CBD Isolate

Some of the distillate is further purified to crystalline CBD. This crystalline, pure material is used to make our CBD Isolate products.

Panacea's Commitment to Research

Having products that are optimally formulated for best effects and delivery mechanisms that ensure maximum benefit are important in this industry and do differentiate our company.

The more data that we have to stand on, the more legitimate we become for the clients we are speaking to, whether this is an end user, physician, veterinarian, retail store or distributor. People are looking for natural alternatives to alleviate conditions, we need to be able to provide better guidance from bona fide sources, or our own research. You will have 100% satisfaction in knowing exactly what you're getting within each Panacea product. Not only does Panacea Life Sciences ensure rigorous on-site testing, but every product also undergoes third-party lab verification to ensure Phyto cannabinoid accuracy, no THC, and the purity of CBD. Our products are tested to ensure critical levels of potency, purity, taste, and color are confirmed by the highest standard of testing available. Before you use cannabidiol (CBD), you should know whether or not the CBD is pure and free of toxins. Good health begins with the purest products. Panacea goes above and beyond in testing our CBD because health begins on subtle levels.

POTENCY TESTING: Potency testing ensures that the cannabinoid level on the label is correct. Proper dosage, whether using as a supplement or for more intense circumstances, is essential. We make sure that testing identifies the amount of CBD, THC and other cannabinoid concentrations in the plant.

RESIDUAL TESTING: A complete lab test should include analyses of the residual solvents. Panacea products contain no solvents; too high concentrations of solvents like ethanol, propane, carbon dioxide or acetone can lead to unpleasant health effects and can turn the products into highly flammable ones.

MICROBE TESTING: Microbiological testing ensures that no harmful bacteria or mold was found in the hemp plant used during the extraction process. These are standard tests that are conducted in the food and dietary supplement industries to ensure products are safe for human or pet consumption. These tests show the product is safe to consume as we ensure there are not harmful yeast, molds or bacteria in the product.

TERPENE TESTING: Terpene testing is essential to understand the levels of terpenes present in the hemp oil ingredient or final product. Terpenes, often overlooked, have unique biological effects that work symbiotically with cannabinoids such as CBD, to provide enhanced health benefits. Terpene testing identifies the range of terpene compounds retained from the Panacea plant at extraction so you can determine whether a product is full-spectrum or isolate.

TOXIN TESTING: Pesticide testing ensures that the hemp compounds used in the extraction process are safe and pesticide free! hemp is sometimes treated with pesticides, potentially causing significant side effects if in high concentrations.

HEAVY METAL TESTING: All products are tested to ensure they are free from heavy metals the hemp plant naturally absorbs from the soil. Metals tested for are Arsenic, Cadmium, Lead, and Mercury.

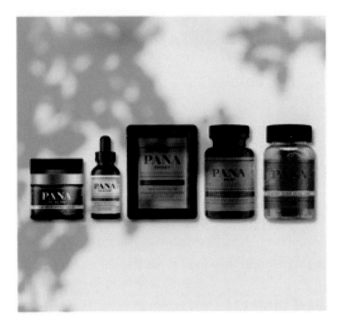

SOLVENT TESTING: A complete lab test should include analyses of the residual solvents. Panacea products contain no solvents; too high concentrations of solvents like ethanol, propane, carbon dioxide or acetone can lead to unpleasant health effects and can turn the products into highly flammable ones.

Our Products

CBD extract is versatile and is easily made or mixed in with other products. As a result, you have many choices when it comes to finding the right one for you.

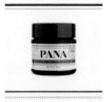

Topicals and Beauty Products

Most CBD topicals include things like lotions, salves, and balms. These are more likely to have a focused, localized effect than they are to have an overall effect (unlike oral CBD products). This is because the CBD never enters the bloodstream with topicals. Instead, the CBD enters through the pores and stays in the area it is applied to do its work.

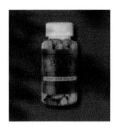

Edibles

You may be able to guess what CBD edibles are. They are any food or drink that has been made with CBD extract. These are very popular as they are easy to take and taste great. However, nothing is perfect and CBD edibles do have their drawback. The edible needs to digest before the CBD can start working, making them the slowest to start working out of all the CBD products. Nonetheless, this is balanced out by the fact that their effect tends to last longer than most products.

Capsules & tablets

Many people prefer their dietary supplements to be more pill-like. If that is you, then there is no need to worry because there are CBD capsules and tablets. CBD capsules are usually soft gels. That means that they have been made with liquid CBD extract. The benefit of soft gels over hard- packed pills is that they tend to digest more quickly, so they start working faster. Similarly, CBD tablets are usually sublingual. This means that you place them under your tongue and allow them to dissolve. The benefit in this is that the skin under your tongue is thin and allows for the CBD to absorb into the system faster.

Oils & tinctures

  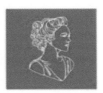

These are one of the simpler and most common kinds of CBD products. They are CBD extract that has been mixed with a carrier oil, like coconut oil. They tend to be rather popular because they provide some flexibility in how you take them. One way is by mixing them in with food or drink. However, like with edibles, you do need to wait for the food or drink to digest before the CBD can start working. The other way is by placing a drop or two directly into your mouth, preferably under your tongue. This is like the sublingual tablets. The thin skin under your tongue lets the CBD absorb quickly.

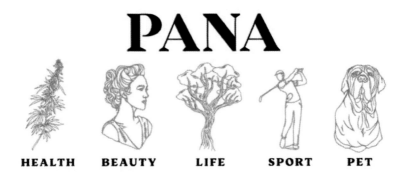

K-tape and Patches

If you are an athlete, you probably already know what K-tape is, as it is fairly common in the athletic world. The more generic name is elastic therapeutic tape, but the more common name is kinesiology (kinesio) tape. It is an elastic cotton bandage made with an adhesive. Its aim is to help deal with the pain that comes from athletic injuries. It was invented in the 1970s by Dr.

Kenzo Kase. He was a chiropractor who was looking for a way to provide his patients with a form of physical support that would not inhibit their movements.

K-tape is popular with pretty much every kind of athlete because it is versatile and can be used for a number of different of reasons. For example, some use it for its initial intended purpose, to help deal with injuries that still allows for movement. Others use it to help support weaker areas of their bodies (for example, supporting your ankle if you

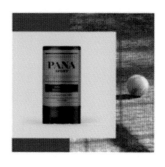

have Achilles tendonitis). Some use it as way to enhance their performance in their chosen sport. <u>Some runners believe it can be used as a way of "'waking up' the muscle."</u> These are just some of these more popular uses, as there are still more that some athletes swear by.

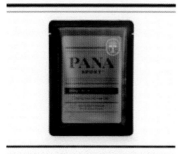

Let's start with CBD on its own. There are many different therapeutic uses for CBD that have be looked at by researchers. One that has been studied a lot is CBD's potential ability to support joint health. For example, <u>this study</u> looked at collagen-induced arthritis in mice. Some of the mice were given CBD, while the rest were given nothing. Those mice that were given the cannabinoid saw a slowing of the spread of the arthritis and lessened damage created by the condition. This study suggests that CBD may be able to support joint health by reducing the damage done by arthritis.

These studies both on K-tape and on CBD suggest that both could provide aid to athletes who are struggling with their joint health. So, it follows that a CBD K-tape may be able to help provide that aid in one fell swoop without the need for several different products. As of right now, there have

70

been no studies that have been done on the combination of CBD and K-tape, but as time goes on, it is likely that we are going to learn more about both and have a better idea of how they work together.

Panacea Life Sciences Now, and into the Future

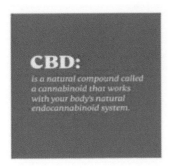

CBD:
is a natural compound called a cannabinoid that works with your body's natural endocannabinoid system.

It is hard to say what exactly the future holds for Panacea Life Sciences, but it does seem exciting. This is mainly due to the fact that Panacea Life Sciences is always developing new products for people and pets (like CBD hand sanitizer, for example). The company also is constantly trying to learn everything there is to know about CBD as they continue to help fund research and do their own.

Whatever promising areas the future has to offer the CBD industry, it is clear to see that Panacea Life Sciences will be at the forefront. It will be worth keeping an eye on this company to see what other developments will come from them.

Panacea Life Sciences has made a serious splash in the CBD industry, and it is not hard to see why when you understand their story. They have shown dedication to producing the highest quality products possible and to helping the world have a better understanding of what CBD is and how it may help people.

What to Look for When Buying Hemp Products

If you perform an internet search for CBD (cannabidiol) oil, you will have millions of results with thousands of companies offering a variety of CBD products for sale . But how do you know which companies are actually worth buying from? There are so many options, it can feel overwhelming trying to weed out the good from the bad.

There are three main CBD extraction methods that manufacturers use to make their products. These are full-spectrum, broad-spectrum, and CBD isolate. The differences between them are based in the other cannabinoids and compounds that are found in the extract with the CBD. Full spectrum has all of the compounds and cannabinoids that come out with the CBD. This includes THC, though the THC content legally cannot be more than 0.3%, which is not enough to create a high.

Broad-spectrum is similar in that it has a majority of the cannabinoids and compounds that the full spectrum has. The one exception is that it does not have any THC. These two are popular options because of something known as the entourage effect. This is where compounds build on each other to create a stronger effect. However, if you are looking for a clearer CBD experience and do not mind it being weaker, then you will want to look for CBD isolate. This kind of extract is exactly what it sounds like. It is just CBD. There are no other compounds or cannabinoids in it.

What to look for in a good CBD company

There are many factors to pay attention to when looking for a good CBD company to buy from. When looking for a reputable CBD company, it's important to do your research. Be sure to read reviews about their products and the company as a whole. These reviews should be both from the company's site and from third party sites. This way you avoid bias and get a clear idea of how good their products really are.

Any trustworthy CBD manufacturer should be as transparent as possible about their processes. They should have their extraction process laid out somewhere on their site for you to read. They should also be open about the rest of their manufacturing process as well. If they do not have this information readily available, then you should stay away.

Reputable CBD companies should also test their products. They should have their testing information available on their site. They should be testing not only the quality of their products, but also to be sure that no unwanted compounds are in the CBD. It is not a problem if they do their own testing, but if they do, they should also have a third-party test their products to be sure that there is no bias in the tests. If they have no information about their testing on their site, you should avoid them.

It also helps to understand what the most recent information that the Food and Drug Administration (FDA) has released on CBD is. If a CBD company is not compliant with what the FDA has laid out or does not even talk about it anywhere on their site, you may want to avoid them. All CBD companies should be keeping up with FDA regulations and guidelines.

Price is another factor you should pay attention to when it comes to high-quality CBD. Some manufacturers charge an exorbitant amount, just because the industry is relatively new, and they feel like they can. This is not an indication as to whether or not the company has quality products. But, on the other end of the spectrum, there are some companies whose prices feel like they are too good to be true. In those cases, they often are. If a CBD product seems dirt cheap (even before it goes on sale or has a coupon), there is a chance that it has been made with synthetic CBD, or the company does not follow safe practices. More often than not, it is best to find products that are a bit more middle of the road in their price. Of course, reading reviews, as talked about above, helps weed out the overpriced and untrustworthy a lot.

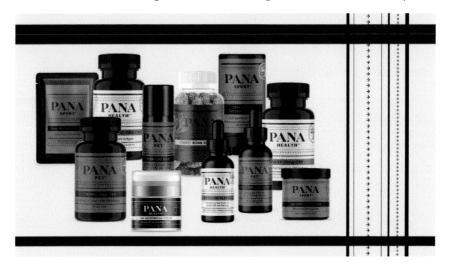

Concluding Remarks

Clearly the emerging regulations, or lack of direction is causing market confusion that is stifling market growth. Farmers are hit with both potential restrictive growing regulations and slowed demand. The lack of progress by the FDA is leading to consumer, manufacturer, and retailer confusion, all of which has needlessly depressed this market. Overall, the hardest hit are consumers who deserve products meeting potency and purity standards as well as proper guidance on how they can gain benefit from these products. We, and others in the hemp industry are urging the regulatory agencies to provide clear and practical regulations to allow the industry to thrive from seed to manufactured products.

DISCLAIMERS:

All information, including statistics, data, claims, etc. are accurate as of July 2020. With the industry's rapid growth, new information is being discovered and updated every day.

All claims made in this book follow the rules and regulations set by the United States Department of Agriculture (USDA).